Firefighter Gary's Fire Safety Rules

Kathleen L. Stone

Dedication

To our Firefighters, EMTs, and Paramedics … 24/7 you are always there in our times of need. Thank you for your sacrifice, thank you for your service!

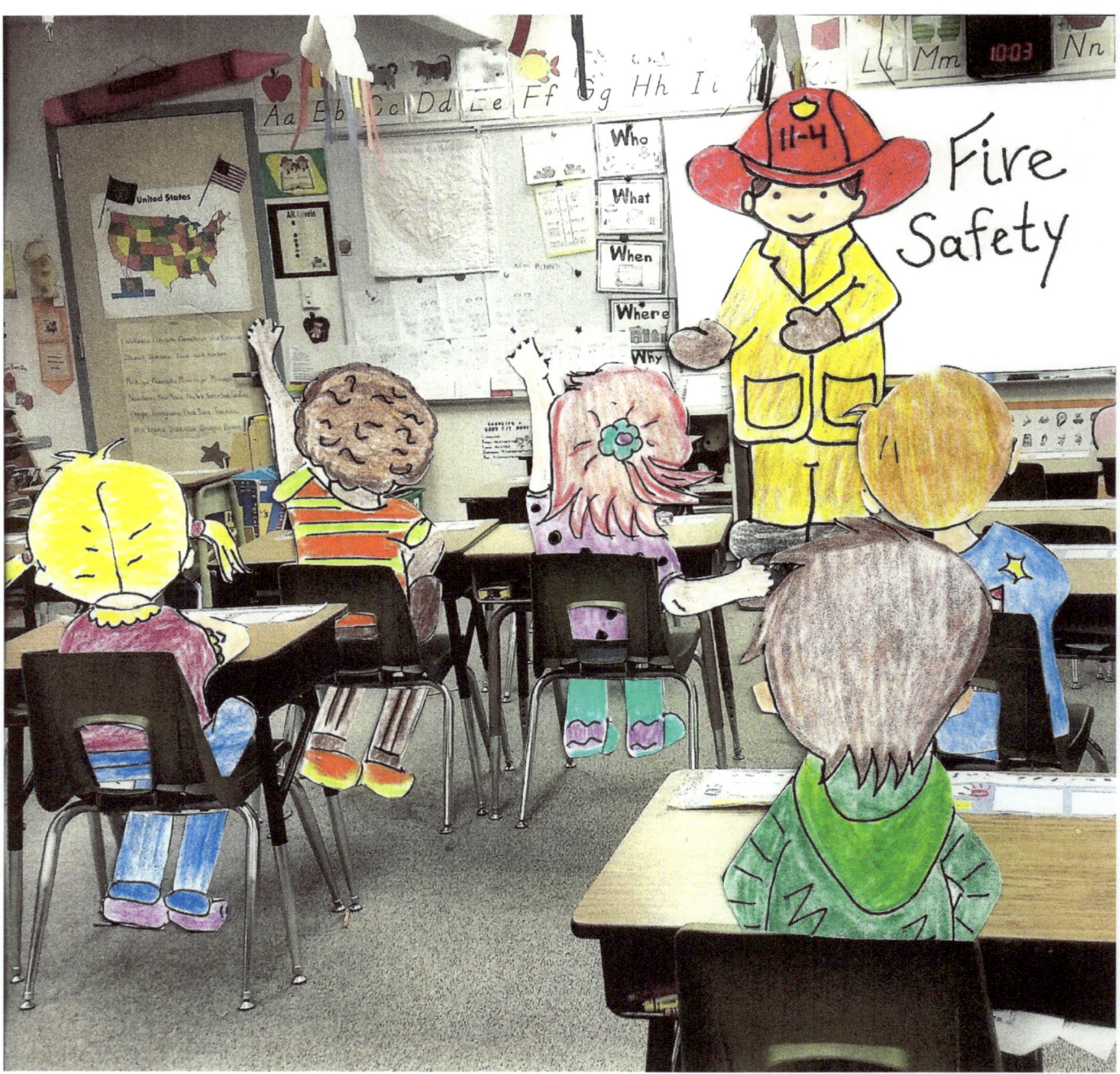

Firefighter Gary
Came to our school
To teach our class
About fire safety rules.

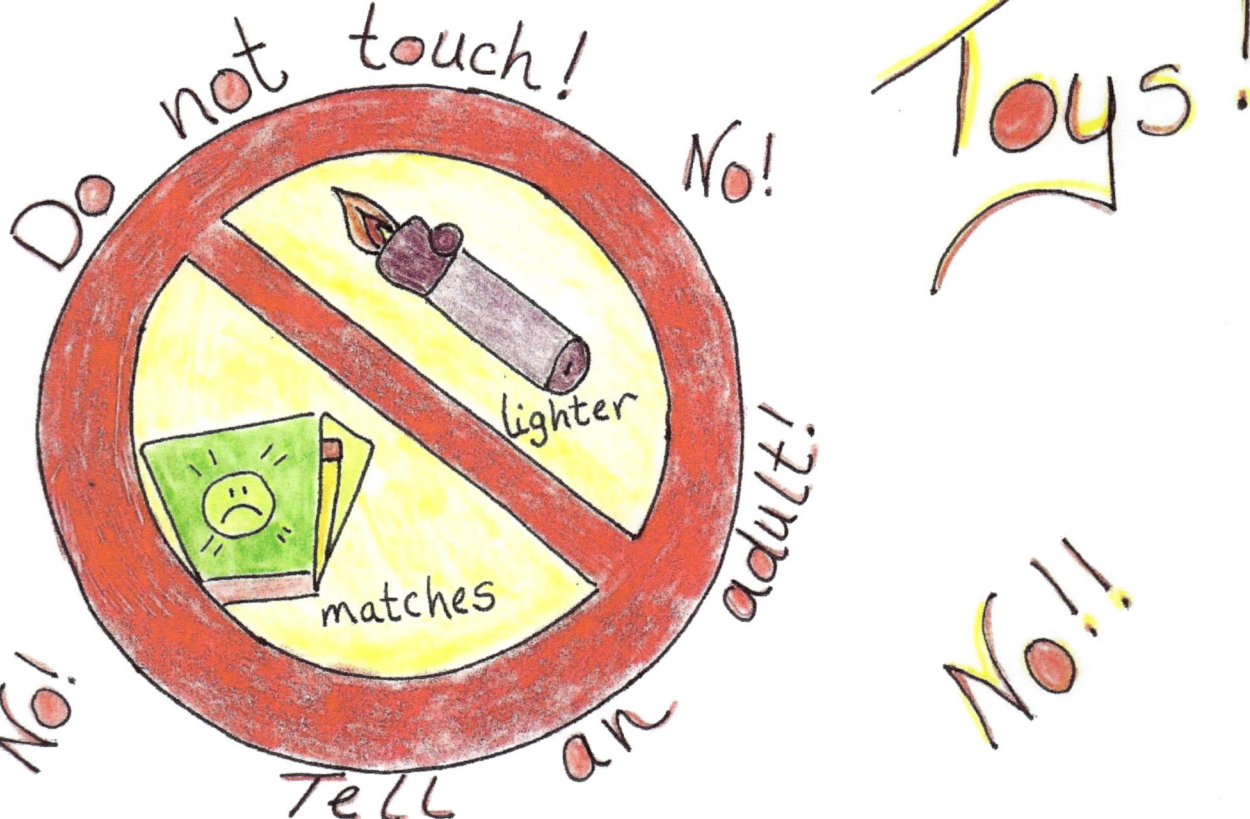

"The most important rule,"
He told the girls and boys,
"Is that matches and lighters
Are not to be played with like toys."

Fire is hot!

Fire moves fast!

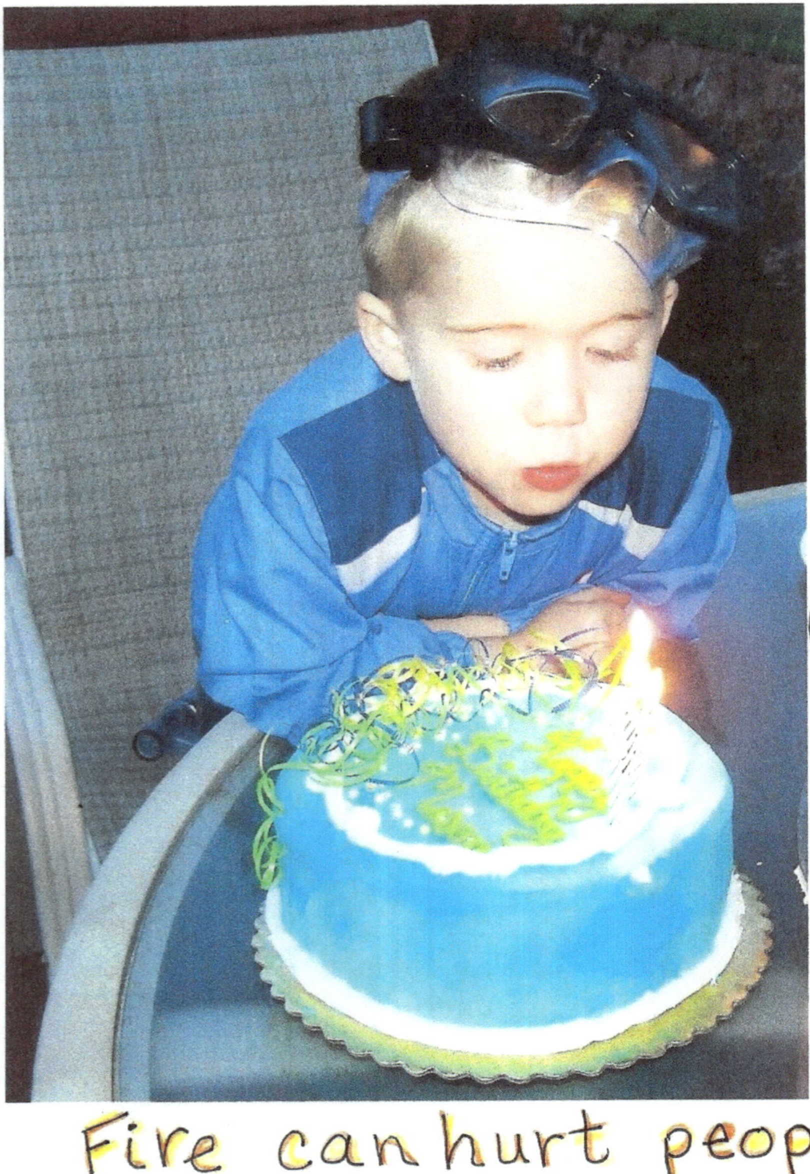

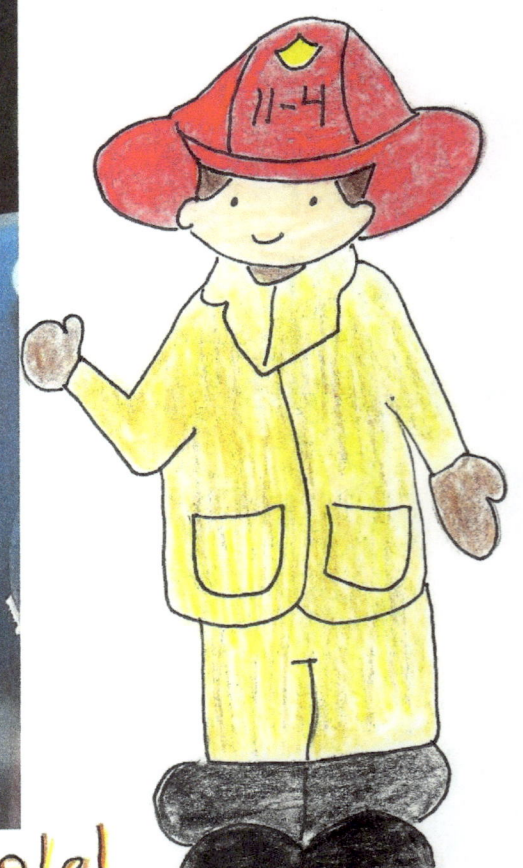

Fire can hurt people!

"Children often make
A serious mistake
Thinking they can put out fires
Like birthday candles on a cake."

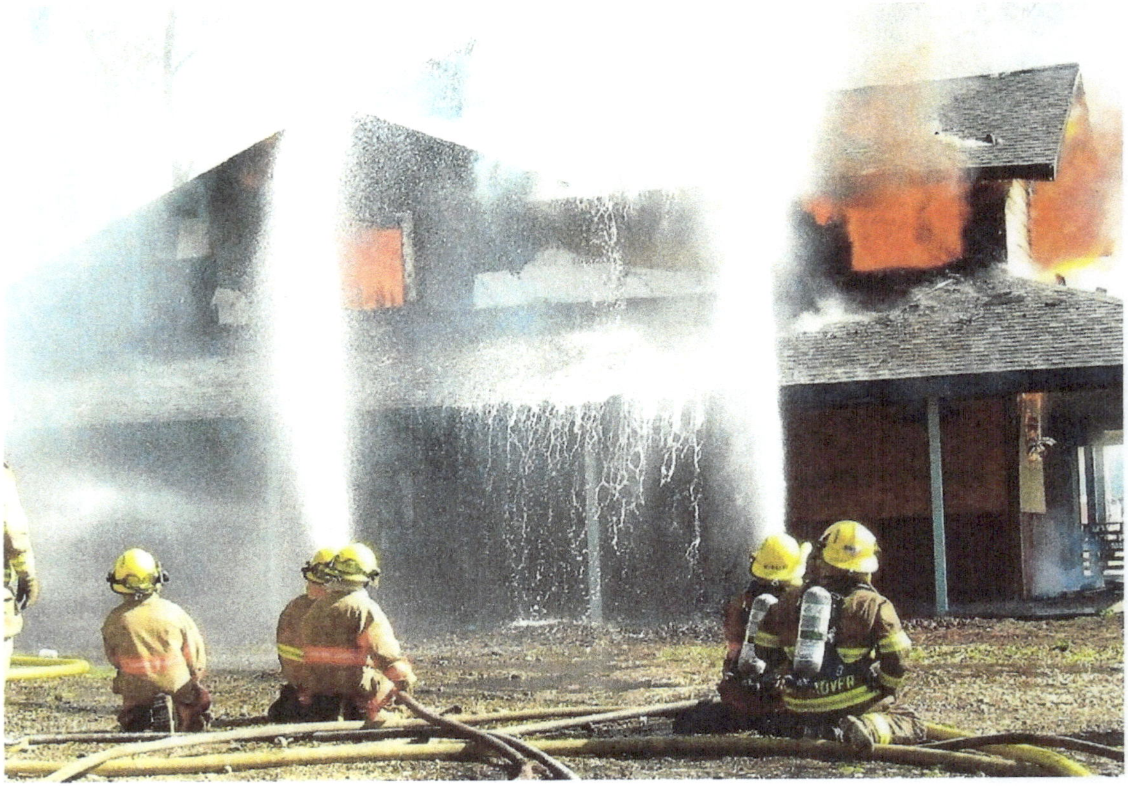

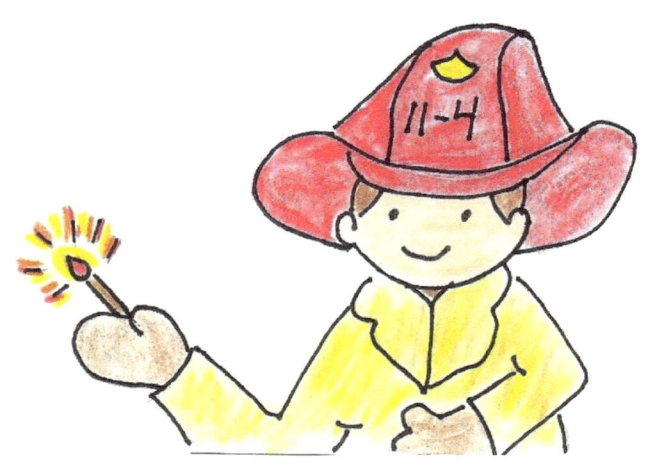

It only takes one tiny flame!

"But fire is fast,
Not something you can tame.
Your whole house can burn
From just one tiny flame."

"Fires hurt people,
Destroying forests, homes, and schools.
So it's important to remember
All these fire safety rules."

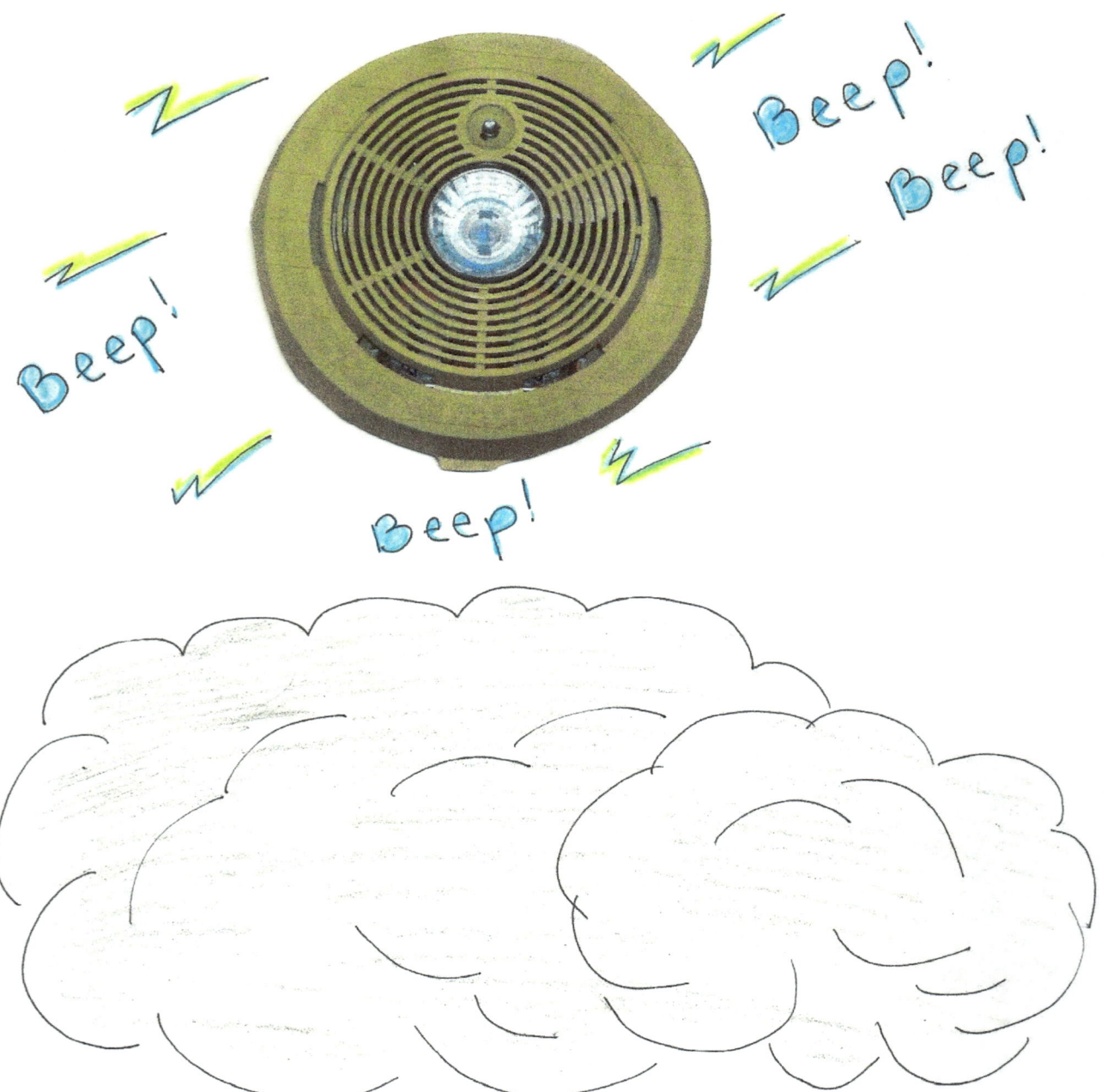

"No matter where you live,
You need smoke detectors all about.
They warn you about fires
And give you time to get out."

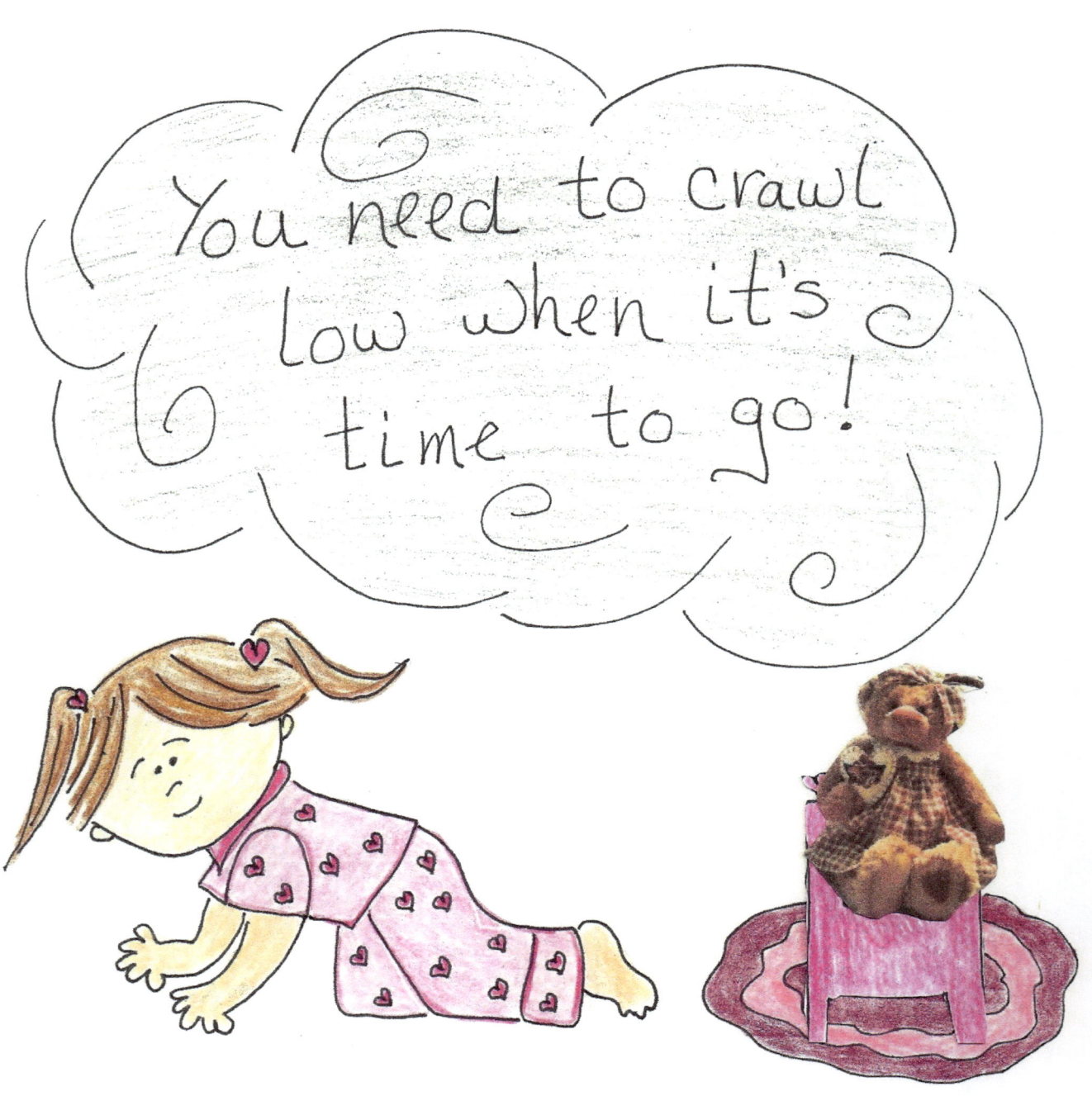

"If your room is full of smoke
Get down low to the ground
Because that's where all the safe
And good air can be found."

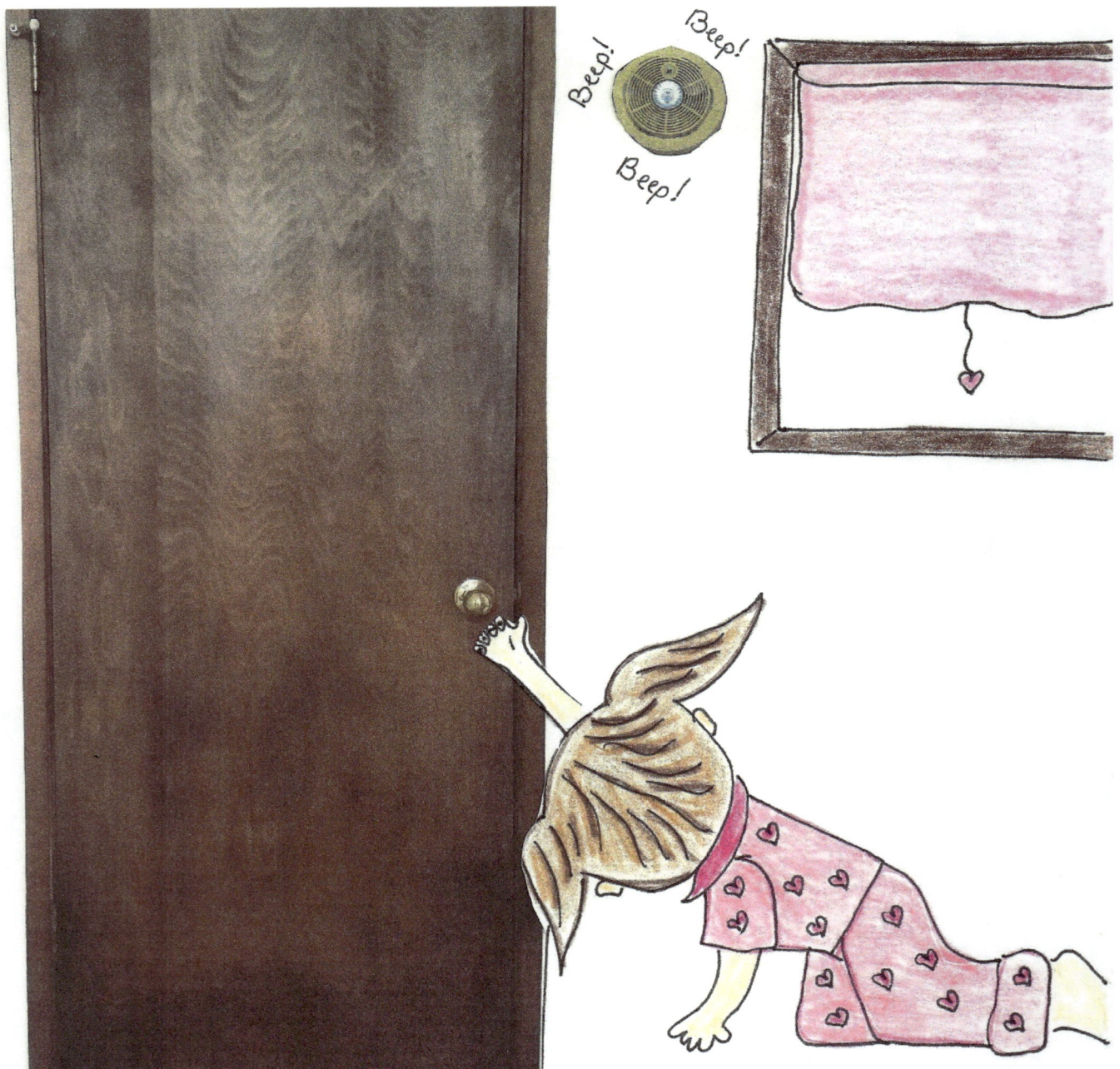

"As soon as you can
Crawl quickly across the floor.
Use the back of your hand and feel
If it's safe to go out the door."

"If your door feels hot,
Find a better way to go.
Remember that fires burn fast
So move quickly, don't be slow!"

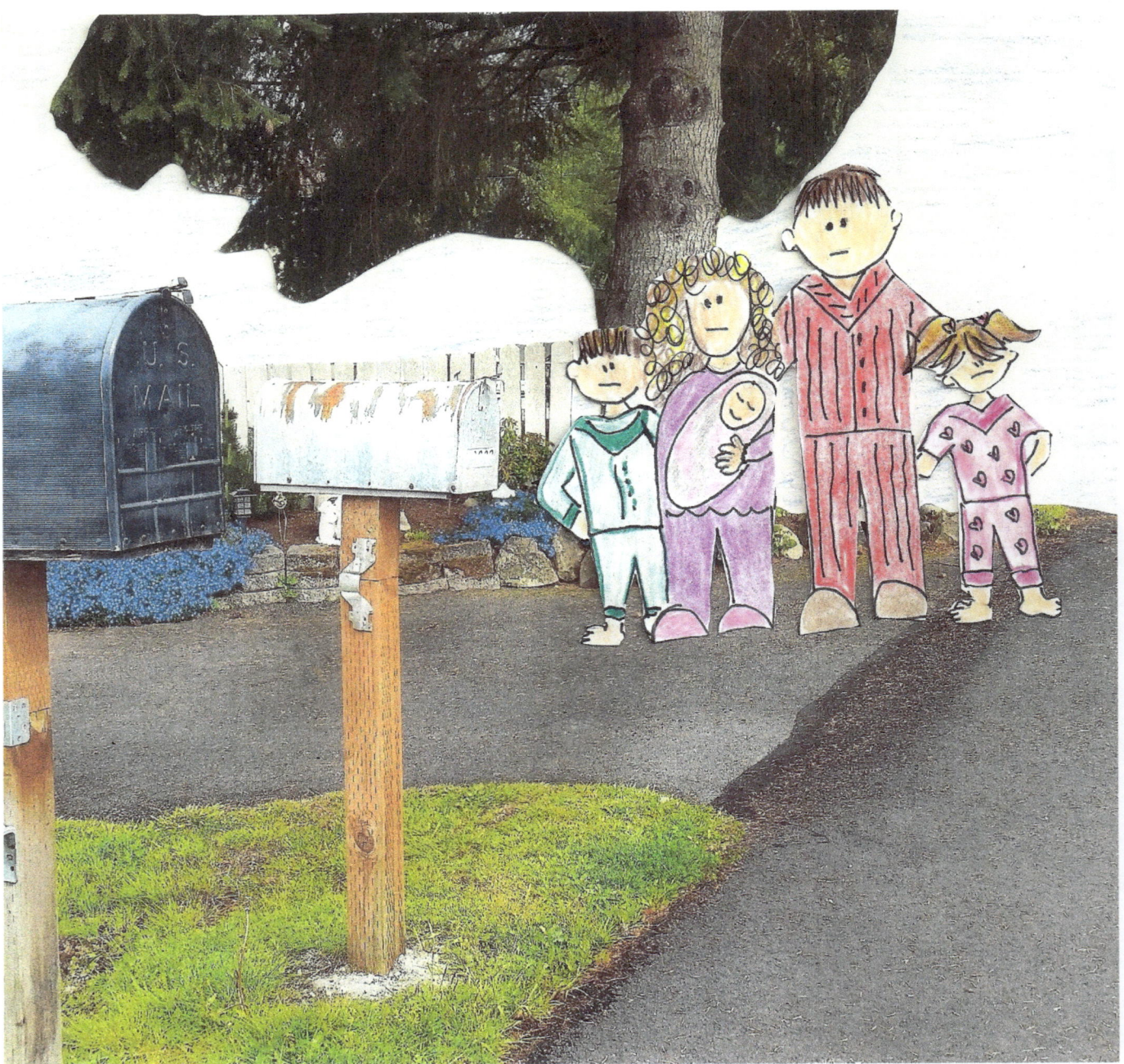

"You might feel scared
But this is not the time to hide.
You will feel much better
When you are safe outside."

"Once you're out, go to a neighbor
And call 911.
Then wait patiently with your family
For the firefighters to come."

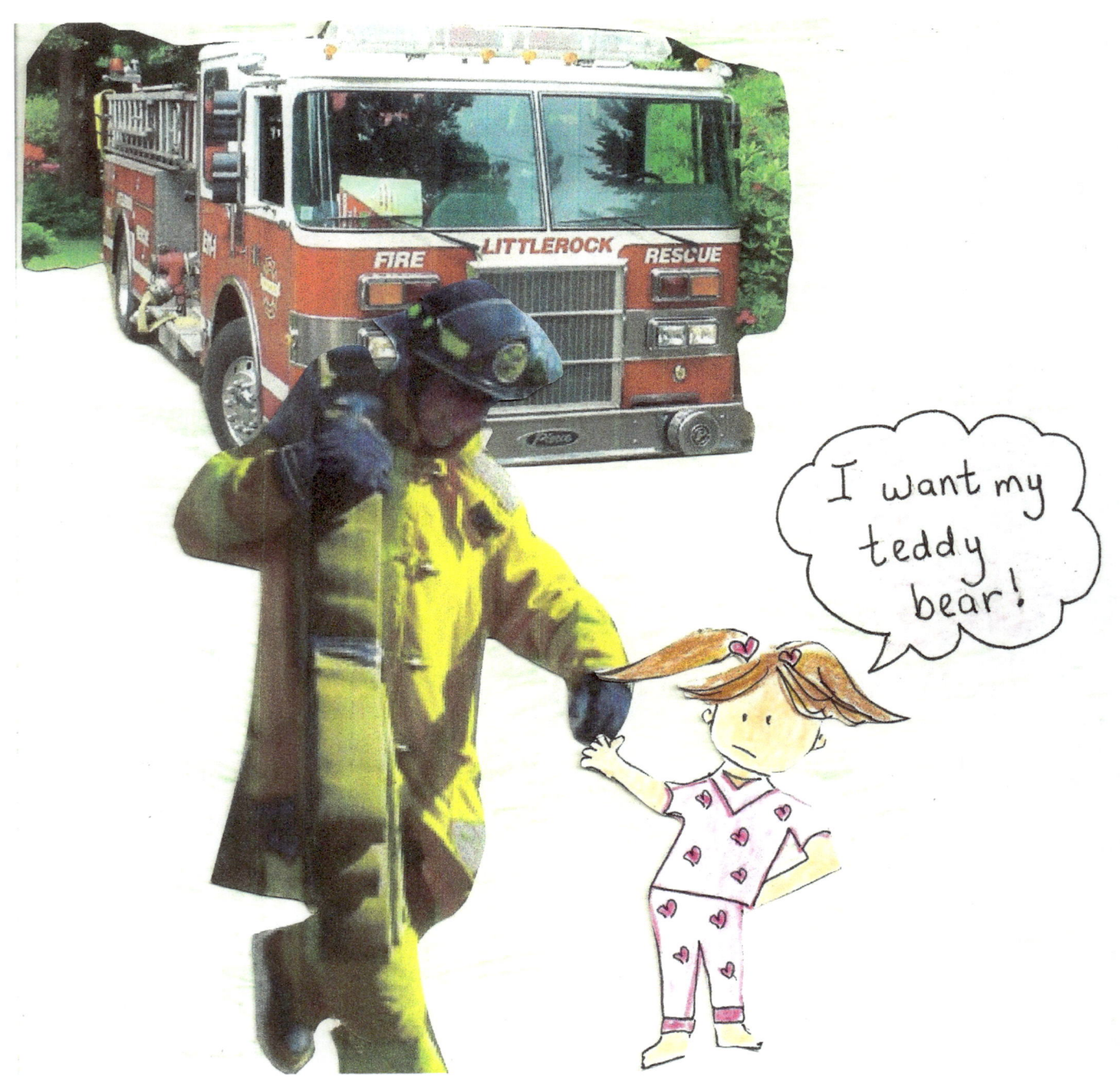

"Now here's another rule
That you should know about.
Never go back in your house for
anything!
YOU NEED TO STAY OUT!"

"Toys can be replaced.
Even pets can too.
Once out, stay out!
Because there's only one you!"

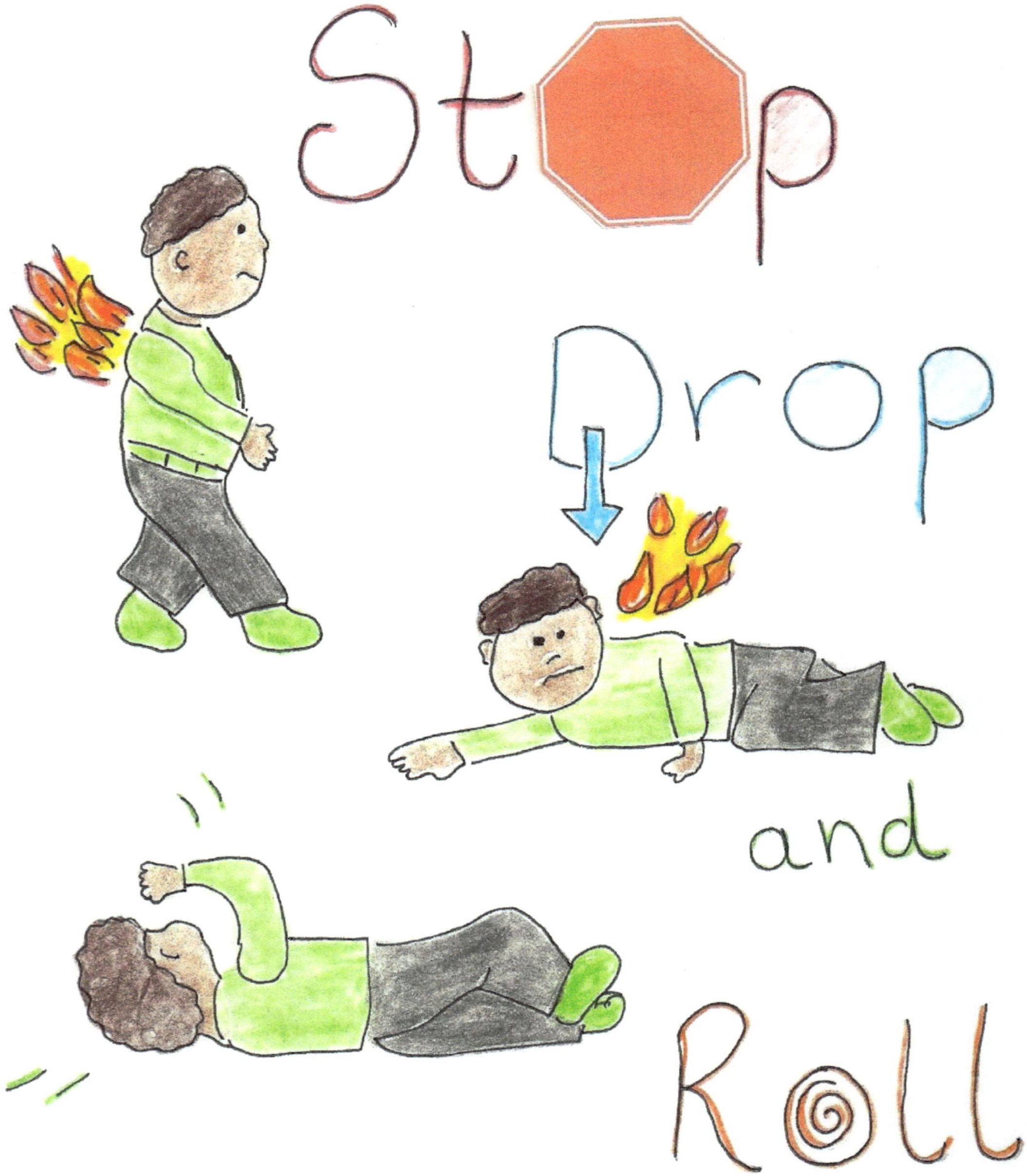
Stop
Drop
and
Roll

"If your clothes should catch on fire
Do not run all about.
STOP, DROP, and ROLL
Until you put the fire out!"

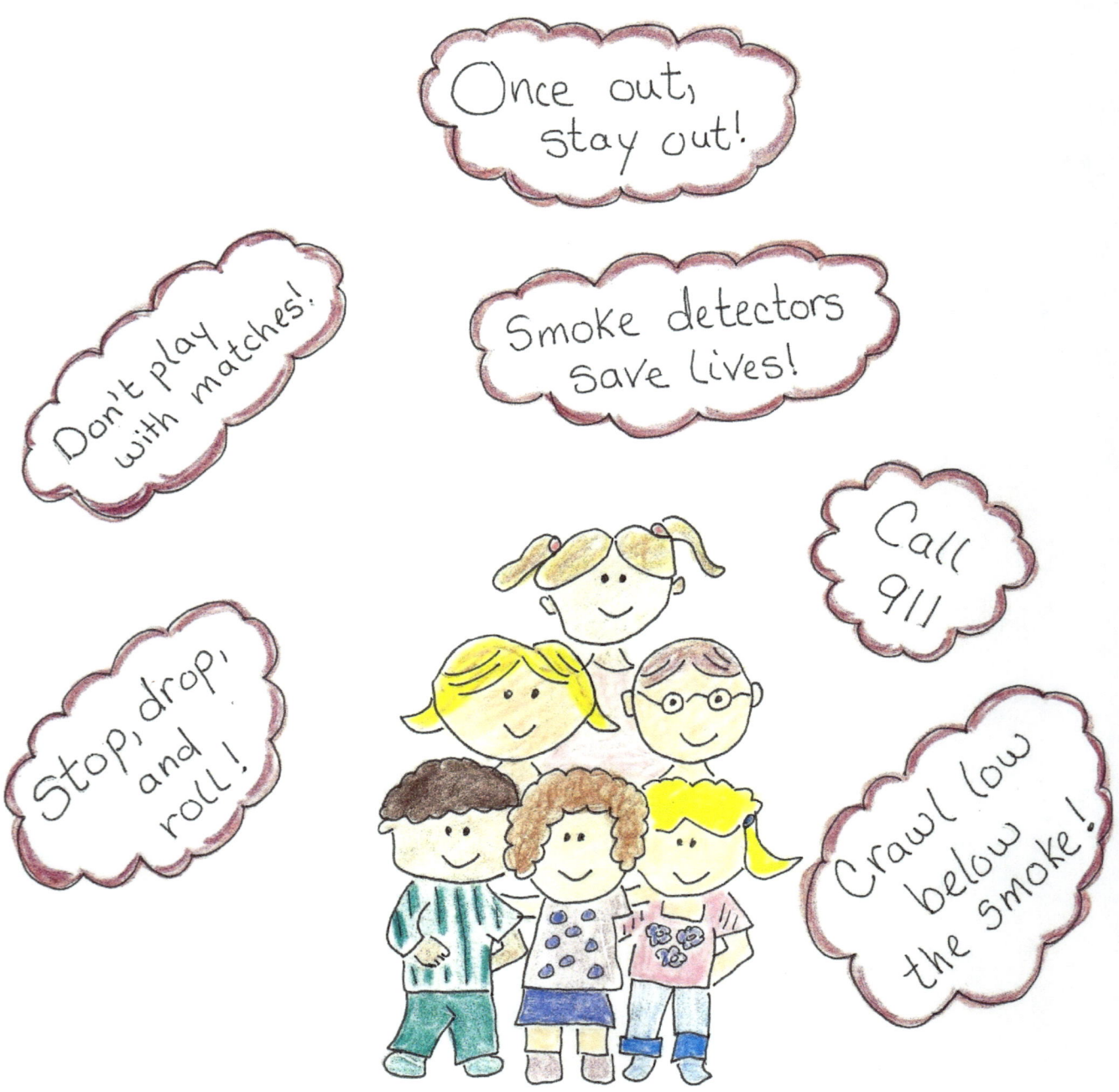

Now we all know the rules
And we will be prepared.
If there ever is a fire
We won't be scared!

Dear Firefighter Gary,

   Thank you for coming to our class and teaching us fire safety rules! We promise to never play with matches or lighters. We will always be safe!

Your friends from
Room 6

Firefighter Gary
Station 11-1

We promised Firefighter Gary
We'd stay safe and be good.
We'll follow all the safety rules
Just like we know we should!

Children and Fire

Fire setting by children is a problem that needs immediate attention. Almost every child has some curiosity about fire. But progression from mere interest in fire to fire play and fire setting can result in devastating destruction, physical injury, and even death. Each year in our country fires set by children result in hundreds of lives lost, thousands of burn injuries, and millions of dollars in property damage. Children make up 15-20% of all fire deaths. Many of those deaths are preschool age children who were simply around the fire setter. It is vital that fire departments work with schools and families to educate children about fire safety and the consequences of fire setting. If you have a child that you suspect is involved in fire setting, please contact your local fire department and ask about their Juvenile Firesetter Intervention program.

Enrichment Activities

ABC's of Fire Safety

Brainstorm phrases for each letter of the alphabet and then assign each child a letter to create a class alphabet book on fire safety. For example, "A is for **always** … **Always** tell an adult if you find matches or lighters, B is for **big** … **Big** fires start small but grow fast, C is for **call** … **Call** 911 from a neighbor's house" etc. Children can write and illustrate their fire safety rule.

Visiting Firefighter

Take a field trip to your local fire department or invite a firefighter to come to your class to discuss fire safety. Important topics to cover include …

- ♥ **Firefighters are our friends. Do not hide from them.**
  This is a great time for children to see the firefighter's clothing and gear.
- ♥ **Do not play with matches or lighters.**
- ♥ **Practice what to do if the smoke alarm goes off.**
  - crawl low to the ground below the smoke (have a child role play this)
  - feel the door from the bottom up with the back of your hand
  - always have two ways out of a room
  - have a prearranged meeting place for your family members
  - once out, stay out … don't go back in for anything
- ♥ **Get out quickly**
  - call 911 from a neighbor's house
  - once out, stay out
- ♥ **Stop, drop, and roll (and cover your face)**
  Have a child demonstrate this.

EDITH (Exit Drills in the Home)

Provide a homework assignment for families to plan and practice fire drills at home. Have them make a floor plan of their home that includes:

- ♥ location of smoke detectors
- ♥ two ways out of each room
- ♥ safety ladders for second floor rooms
- ♥ the location of their meeting place away from their home

More Fire Safety Resources

You can find lots of free resources and lesson plan ideas online. Your local fire department should have additional resources and materials for you as well. They would also be a great resource for information on how to put on your own safety fair at school.

ABOUT THE AUTHOR

Kathleen L. Stone is a National Board Certified educator with over thirty-five years teaching experience. She is currently teaching second grade with North Thurston Public Schools in Washington State. Mrs. Stone and her husband, Gary, are also *Juvenile Firesetter Interventionists* with West Thurston Regional Fire. Together they work with children, ages 3-16, and their families that have been involved in fire setting situations. The program not only teaches children about fire safety, but also focuses on the dangers and consequences of fire setting.

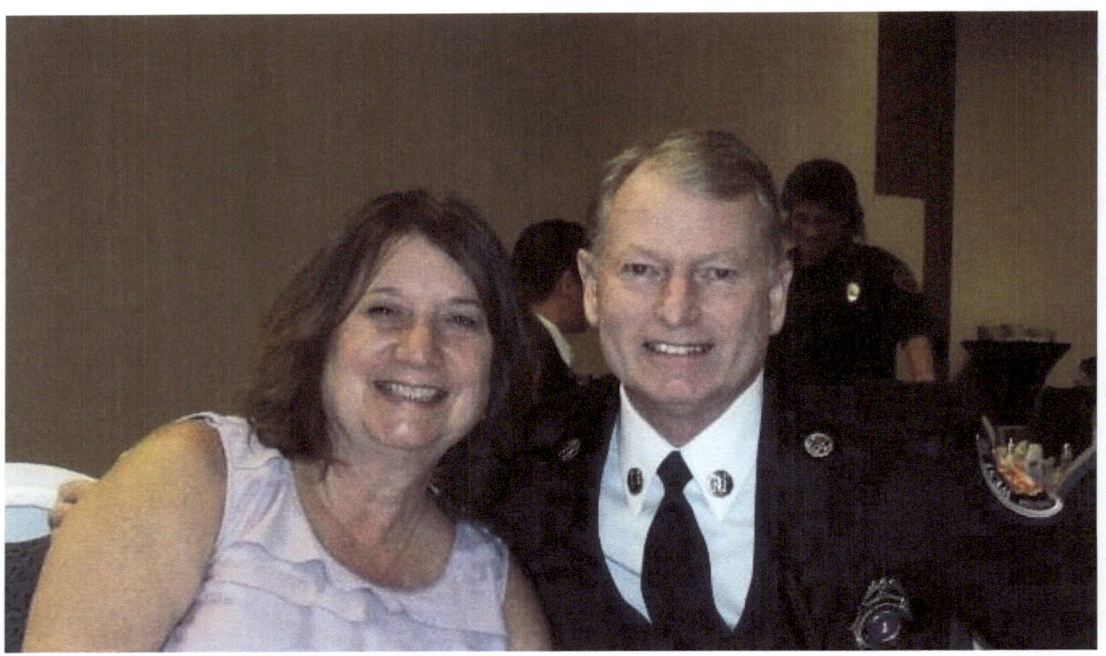

Enjoy these other books by Kathleen L. Stone

Penguin Place Value
A Math Adventure

Number Line Fun
Solving Number Mysteries

Riley the Robot
An Input/Output Machine

Mason the Magician
Hundreds Chart Addition

Katelyn's Fair Share Picnic
More Math Fun

Money Tree Mysteries
Adventures with Quarters

Alien Even and Alien Odd
A Math Space Adventure

Kenley's Line Plot Graph
Another Math Adventure

Matthew's Sunshine Bakery
Multiplication Arrays

From My Quilted Heart to Yours
Heart Warming Quilts and Heart Healthy Recipes for Your Loved Ones